The Ultimate Weight Loss Solution:

Discovering the Secret to Sustainable Health and Happiness

By

Ismael A. Fisher

Table of Contents

<u>Chapter 3: Exercise</u>

The Key to Boosting Metabolism and Burning Fat.
The benefits of regular exercise for weight loss and overall health.
Types of exercise and their impact on metabolism.
Tips for designing an effective exercise program.
The importance of movement and staying active throughout the day.

<u>Chapter 4: Lifestyle Factors</u>

The Importance of Sleep, Stress Management, and Mindfulness.
The role of sleep in weight loss and overall health.
Understanding stress and its impact on weight.

Mindfulness and its role in healthy eating and weight loss.
Other lifestyle factors that impact weight, such as smoking and alcohol consumption

<u>Chapter 5: Setting Goals and Staying Motivated</u>

Introduction:

Welcome to "The Secret to Ultimate Weight Loss," a book that aims to provide you with the tools and knowledge you need to achieve sustainable weight loss and improve your overall health and well-being. Losing weight can be a challenging and complex journey, but with the right approach and mindset, it can also be an empowering and rewarding one.

In this book, we'll explore the latest research and insights into weight loss, including the importance of nutrition, exercise, and lifestyle factors. You'll discover practical strategies and tips for setting achievable goals, staying motivated, and overcoming common obstacles along the way.

Whether you're just starting your weight loss journey or looking to take your efforts to the next level, this book will provide you with the knowledge and inspiration you need to succeed. So let's get started on unlocking the secret to ultimate weight loss together.

Chapter 1: Introduction

The Importance of Sustainable Weight Loss

Sustainable weight loss is the process of losing weight in a manner that is healthy and maintainable over the long term. Unlike crash diets or extreme weight loss measures, sustainable weight loss focuses on making gradual, lasting changes to one's diet, exercise habits, and overall lifestyle. It is an approach that promotes not only weight loss but also overall health and well-being, and it is considered the most effective way to achieve and maintain a healthy weight.

The importance of sustainable weight loss cannot be overstated, as excess body weight has been linked to a variety of health problems, including heart disease, diabetes, and cancer. Losing weight and maintaining a healthy weight can significantly reduce the risk of developing these and other chronic health conditions.

Additionally, sustainable weight loss has been shown to improve mental health and quality of life. Losing excess weight can boost self-esteem, improve mood, and increase energy levels, all of which contribute to a better overall sense of well-being.

One of the key benefits of sustainable weight loss is that it promotes healthy habits that can be maintained over the long term. Instead of relying on extreme diets or exercise regimens that are unsustainable, sustainable weight loss emphasizes making gradual changes that are achievable and sustainable. This approach not only leads to weight loss but also helps individuals develop healthier habits that can be maintained over the long term.

Furthermore, sustainable weight loss is more likely to lead to long-term success than crash diets or extreme weight loss measures. These approaches may result in rapid weight loss in the short term, but they are often unsustainable and can lead to weight gain once the diet or exercise regimen is discontinued. Sustainable weight loss, on the other hand, focuses on making lasting changes that can be maintained over time, leading to long-term weight loss success.

In summary, sustainable weight loss is essential for overall health and well-being. It promotes healthy habits that can be maintained over the long term, leading to lasting weight loss and a better overall quality of life. By focusing on making gradual, maintainable changes to one's diet, exercise habits, and overall lifestyle, individuals can achieve and maintain a healthy weight and reduce the risk of chronic health conditions.

Understanding the consequences of being overweight

Being overweight or obese can have numerous negative consequences on an individual's health, both in the short and long term. Some of the most significant consequences of being overweight include:

Increased risk of chronic diseases: Being overweight is a significant risk factor for several chronic diseases, including heart disease, diabetes, high blood pressure, stroke, and certain types of cancer. These diseases can be life-threatening and can significantly impact an individual's quality of life.

Cardiovascular problems: Excess weight puts additional strain on the heart, leading to an increased risk of heart disease, heart attack, and stroke.

Joint problems: Being overweight can put additional stress on the joints, leading to joint pain, arthritis, and an increased risk of joint injuries.

Sleep apnea: Sleep apnea is a condition in which an individual's breathing repeatedly stops and starts during sleep. Being overweight is a significant risk factor for sleep apnea, which can cause daytime fatigue, headaches, and other health problems.

Mental health problems: Being overweight can also have negative effects on mental health, including low self-esteem, depression, and anxiety.

Reduced life expectancy: Studies have shown that being overweight or obese can shorten an individual's lifespan. The excess weight can increase the risk of developing chronic diseases, which can ultimately lead to premature death.

In addition to these health consequences, being overweight can also impact an individual's daily life. It can lead to decreased mobility, difficulty with physical activities, and a reduced quality of life overall.

In conclusion, being overweight can have severe consequences on an individual's health and well-being. It is essential to maintain a healthy weight through regular exercise, a balanced diet, and other healthy lifestyle choices to reduce the risk of chronic diseases and other negative health outcomes.

The benefits of achieving and maintaining a healthy weight

Achieving and maintaining a healthy weight is crucial for overall health and well-being. It can have numerous positive benefits for individuals, including:

Reduced risk of chronic diseases: Maintaining a healthy weight can significantly reduce the risk of developing chronic diseases such as heart disease, diabetes, high blood pressure, stroke, and certain types of cancer.

Improved cardiovascular health: A healthy weight can lead to improved cardiovascular health, including lower blood pressure, reduced risk of heart disease, and improved blood sugar levels.

Increased energy and mobility: Maintaining a healthy weight can improve energy levels and mobility, making it easier to participate in physical activities and everyday tasks.

Improved mental health: A healthy weight can improve mental health, including increased self-esteem, reduced risk of depression and anxiety, and improved overall well-being.

Better sleep: Achieving and maintaining a healthy weight can lead to improved sleep quality, reducing the risk of sleep disorders such as sleep apnea.

Longer lifespan: Studies have shown that maintaining a healthy weight can lead to a longer lifespan, reducing the risk of premature death.

Reduced healthcare costs: Maintaining a healthy weight can reduce healthcare costs associated with chronic diseases and other weight-related health problems.

Overall, achieving and maintaining a healthy weight is essential for a healthy and happy life. It can lead to numerous positive health outcomes, including a reduced risk of chronic diseases, improved cardiovascular health, increased energy and mobility, improved mental health, better sleep, and a longer lifespan. By making healthy lifestyle choices such as regular exercise and a balanced diet, individuals can achieve and maintain a healthy weight and enjoy these many benefits.

Why sustainable weight loss is key to long-term health and happiness

Sustainable weight loss is key to long-term health and happiness because it involves making healthy lifestyle choices that can be maintained over time. It is not just about losing weight quickly through fad diets or extreme measures but about creating sustainable habits that promote overall health and well-being.

Here are some reasons why sustainable weight loss is crucial for long-term health and happiness:

Sustainable weight loss promotes long-term weight management: Sustainable weight loss involves making healthy lifestyle choices that can be maintained over time. This approach promotes long-term weight management, which is essential for maintaining good health and reducing the risk of chronic diseases.

Sustainable weight loss is better for overall health: Rapid weight loss can lead to muscle loss and a slower metabolism, which can make it more difficult to maintain weight loss over time. Sustainable weight loss, on the other hand, involves gradual weight loss through healthy lifestyle changes, which can improve overall health and well-being.

Sustainable weight loss leads to better mental health: Fad diets and extreme weight loss measures can be stressful and have negative effects on mental health. Sustainable weight loss, on the other hand, promotes positive habits that can reduce stress and improve overall mental health.

Sustainable weight loss promotes better eating habits: Sustainable weight loss involves making healthy choices and developing better eating habits, which can lead to improved nutrition and better overall health.

Sustainable weight loss leads to increased self-esteem and confidence: Achieving sustainable weight loss through healthy lifestyle choices can lead to increased self-esteem and confidence, improving overall happiness and well-being.

Chapter 2: Nutrition

The Foundation of Weight Loss

The foundation of weight loss is based on the principle of achieving a calorie deficit. A calorie deficit occurs when an individual burns more calories than they consume through their diet. This causes the body to use stored fat as energy, leading to weight loss.

The foundation of weight loss can be achieved through several strategies:

- Diet modification: One of the most effective ways to achieve a calorie deficit is through modifying one's diet. This can be done by reducing portion sizes, cutting out high-calorie foods, and replacing them with healthier options such as fruits and vegetables.
- Regular exercise: Regular exercise can help burn calories and promote weight

loss. This can include cardio workouts such as running or cycling, as well as strength training exercises to build muscle mass and increase metabolism.

- Lifestyle changes: Small lifestyle changes such as taking the stairs instead of the elevator, walking or cycling to work, or standing instead of sitting can all help to increase daily physical activity and promote weight loss.

- Mindful eating: Mindful eating involves paying attention to hunger and fullness cues and eating slowly and intentionally. This can help individuals make healthier choices and avoid overeating.

It is important to note that weight loss should be achieved in a healthy and sustainable way. Rapid weight loss through extreme measures or fad diets can be harmful to health and may result in weight regain over time. Instead, a gradual and sustainable approach that promotes healthy habits and lifestyle changes is recommended.

In summary, the foundation of weight loss is based on achieving a calorie deficit through diet modification, regular exercise, lifestyle changes, and mindful eating. By adopting healthy and sustainable habits, individuals can achieve and maintain a healthy weight, promoting overall health and well-being.

The basics of nutrition and metabolism

Nutrition and metabolism are closely linked and play a crucial role in overall health and well-being. Nutrition refers to the study of how food affects the body and provides the necessary nutrients for growth, development, and maintenance of bodily functions. Metabolism, on the other hand, refers to the chemical processes that occur in the body to convert food into energy.

The basics of nutrition involve understanding the different macronutrients and micronutrients required for a healthy diet. Macronutrients include carbohydrates, proteins, and fats, while micronutrients include vitamins and minerals. These nutrients are essential for proper growth and development, maintenance of bodily functions, and prevention of chronic diseases.

Carbohydrates provide the body with energy and are found in foods such as grains, fruits, and vegetables. Proteins are necessary for building and repairing tissues and are found in foods such as meat, fish, and beans. Fats provide energy and help to absorb vitamins and minerals, and are found in foods such as nuts, seeds, and oils.

In addition to macronutrients, micronutrients are also essential for overall health. Vitamins and minerals are necessary for many bodily functions such as immune system function, bone health, and energy production.

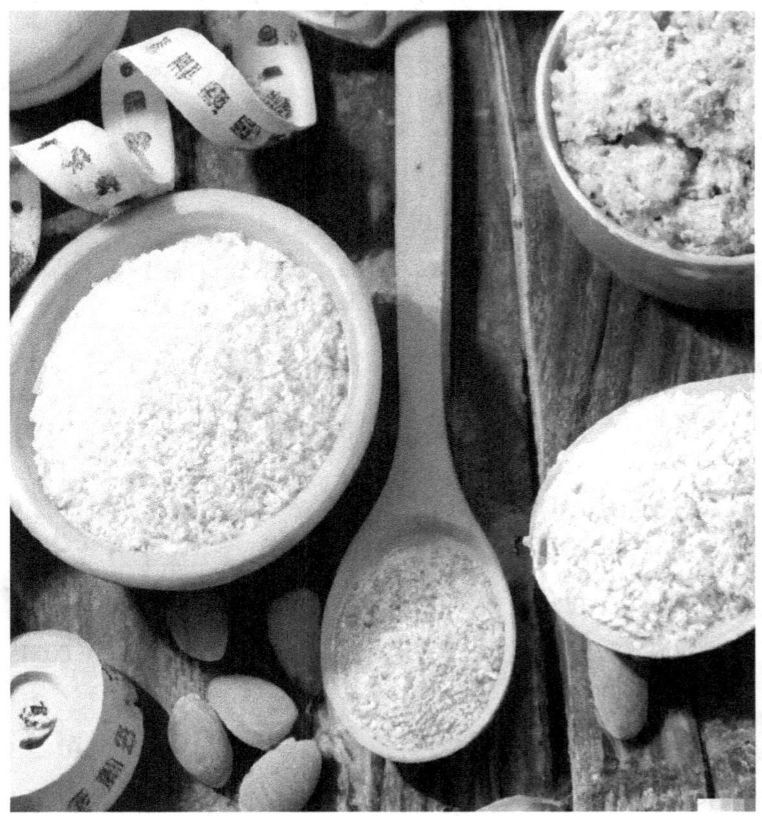

Metabolism is the process by which the body converts food into energy. The body requires energy for all bodily functions, including breathing, digestion, and circulation. Metabolism can be influenced by several factors, including genetics, age, gender, and body composition.

The metabolic rate is the amount of energy the body uses to carry out its functions. A higher metabolic rate can help individuals burn more calories and promote weight loss. Regular exercise and strength training can help to increase the metabolic rate and promote weight loss.

In summary, nutrition and metabolism play a crucial role in overall health and well-being. Understanding the basics of nutrition, including the different macronutrients and micronutrients, and their roles in the body can help individuals make healthier food choices. Understanding metabolism and how it can be influenced by lifestyle factors can also help individuals to achieve and maintain a healthy weight.

Understanding macronutrients and micronutrients

Macronutrients and micronutrients are essential components of a healthy diet. Macronutrients are nutrients required in large quantities and include carbohydrates, proteins, and fats. Micronutrients, on the other hand, are required in smaller quantities and include vitamins and minerals.

Carbohydrates:

Carbohydrates are the body's primary source of energy and are found in foods such as grains, fruits, and vegetables. Carbohydrates can be further divided into simple carbohydrates and complex carbohydrates. Simple carbohydrates, such as those found in candy and sugary drinks, are quickly broken down by the body, leading to a spike in blood sugar levels. Complex carbohydrates, such as those found in whole grains, are broken down more slowly, providing sustained energy.

Protein:

Proteins are essential for building and repairing tissues, as well as for maintaining a healthy immune system. Proteins are found in foods such as meat, fish, beans, and nuts.

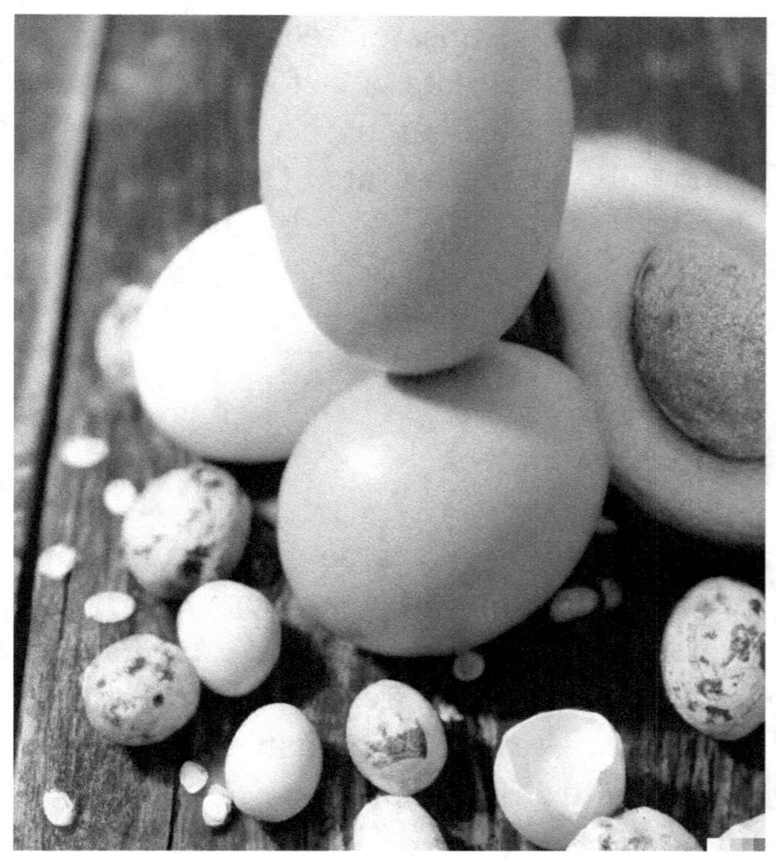

Fats:

Fats are essential for many bodily functions, including energy production and hormone regulation. Fats can be further divided into saturated fats, unsaturated fats, and trans fats. Saturated fats are found in animal products and should be consumed in moderation. Unsaturated fats, found in foods such as nuts, seeds, and oils, are healthier options. Trans fats should be avoided as they have been linked to several health problems.

Micronutrients:

Micronutrients include vitamins and minerals that are necessary for many bodily functions. Vitamins are organic compounds that the body requires in small amounts, while minerals are inorganic compounds required in small amounts.

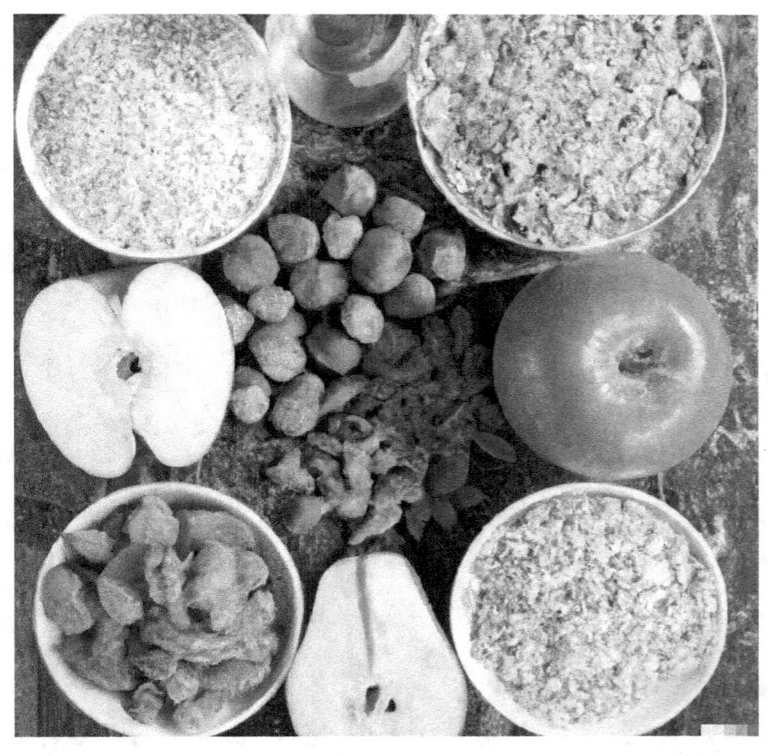

Some examples of vitamins include vitamin C, found in fruits and vegetables, and vitamin D, found in dairy products and sunlight. Some examples of minerals include iron, found in meats and leafy green vegetables, and calcium, found in dairy products.

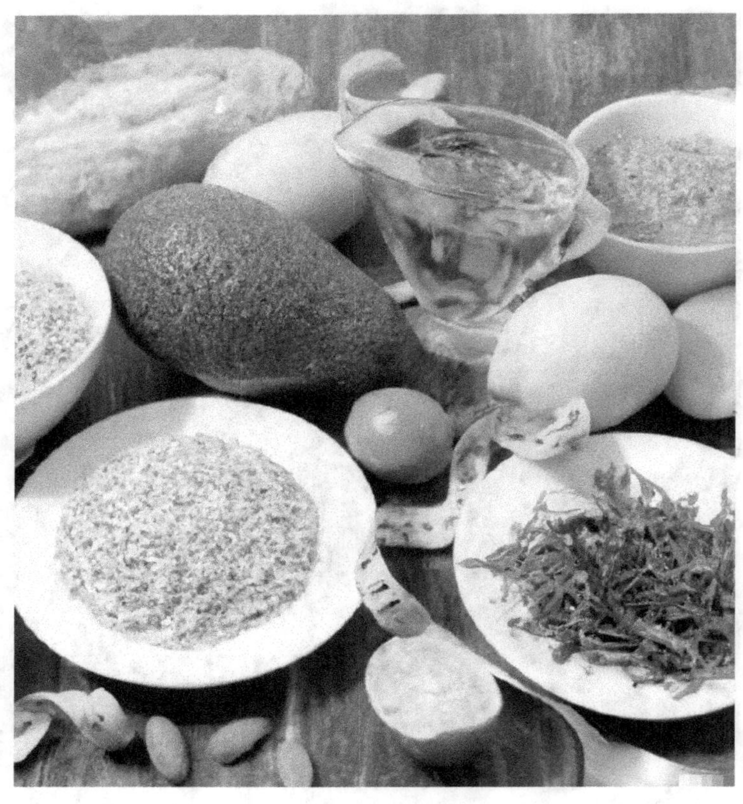

In summary, understanding macronutrients and micronutrients is important for maintaining a healthy and balanced diet. A diet that includes a variety of foods from all macronutrient and micronutrient groups can help to ensure that the body is getting all the nutrients it needs for optimal health and well-being.

The role of diet in weight loss and maintenance

The role of diet in weight loss and maintenance cannot be overstated. In order to lose weight, individuals must consume fewer calories than they burn through physical activity and daily bodily functions. This can be achieved through a combination of reducing calorie intake and increasing physical activity levels.

To reduce calorie intake, individuals can focus on making healthier food choices, such as choosing whole grains instead of refined grains, consuming lean protein sources, and increasing their intake of fruits and vegetables. In addition, reducing portion sizes can also help to reduce calorie intake.

Meal planning and preparation tips for healthy eating

Meal planning and preparation can also play an important role in achieving and maintaining a healthy weight. Here are some tips for healthy eating:

- ☐ Plan ahead: Plan meals and snacks in advance to ensure that healthy options are available when hunger strikes.
- ☐ Shop smart: Stock up on healthy foods and avoid buying unhealthy options that may be tempting.
- ☐ Portion control: Use smaller plates and containers to help control portion sizes.
- ☐ Cook at home: Cooking at home allows individuals to control the ingredients and preparation methods, making it easier to choose healthier options.
- ☐ Include a variety of foods: Eating a variety of foods can help ensure that

the body is getting all the necessary nutrients for optimal health.

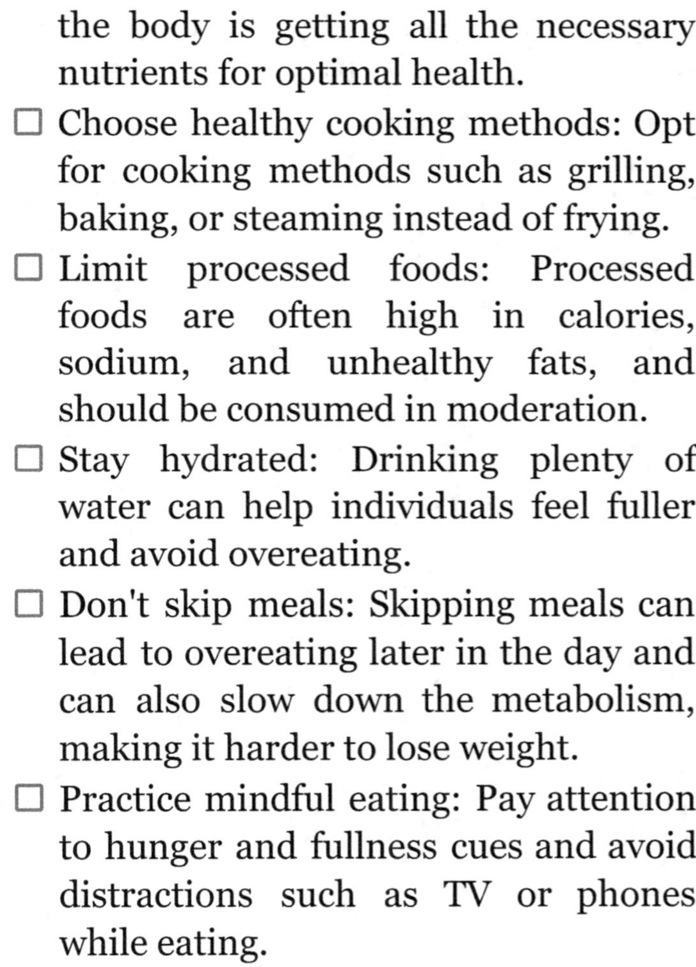

- ☐ Choose healthy cooking methods: Opt for cooking methods such as grilling, baking, or steaming instead of frying.
- ☐ Limit processed foods: Processed foods are often high in calories, sodium, and unhealthy fats, and should be consumed in moderation.
- ☐ Stay hydrated: Drinking plenty of water can help individuals feel fuller and avoid overeating.
- ☐ Don't skip meals: Skipping meals can lead to overeating later in the day and can also slow down the metabolism, making it harder to lose weight.
- ☐ Practice mindful eating: Pay attention to hunger and fullness cues and avoid distractions such as TV or phones while eating.

In summary, the role of diet in weight loss and maintenance is crucial. Healthy eating habits, including meal planning and preparation, can help individuals make healthier food choices and achieve and maintain a healthy weight.

Chapter 3: Exercise

Key to Boosting Metabolism and Burning Fat

The key to boosting metabolism and burning fat is to maintain a healthy diet and engage in regular physical activity. Here are some tips for boosting metabolism and burning fat:

Eat protein-rich foods: Protein has a higher thermic effect than other macronutrients, meaning that the body burns more calories to digest it. Consuming protein-rich foods such as lean meats, fish, and beans can help to boost metabolism.

Drink plenty of water: Drinking water can help to increase metabolism and reduce calorie intake by promoting feelings of fullness.

Engage in strength training: Strength training can help to build muscle mass, which can increase metabolism and help to burn fat.

Get enough sleep: Lack of sleep can disrupt metabolism and lead to weight gain. Getting enough sleep can help to regulate metabolism and promote fat burning.

Consume healthy fats: Healthy fats, such as those found in nuts, seeds, and oils, can help to boost metabolism and promote fat burning.

Stay active throughout the day: Engaging in regular physical activity throughout the day, such as taking the stairs instead of the elevator or going for a walk during lunch breaks, can help to boost metabolism and burn fat.

Eat a balanced diet: Consuming a balanced diet that includes a variety of foods from all macronutrient and micronutrient groups can help to support metabolism and promote fat burning.

Limit processed foods: Processed foods are often high in calories, unhealthy fats, and sugar, and can contribute to weight gain. Limiting processed foods and opting for whole, nutrient-dense foods can help to boost metabolism and promote fat burning.

In summary, boosting metabolism and burning fat requires a combination of healthy eating habits and regular physical activity. By incorporating these tips into a healthy lifestyle, individuals can improve metabolism and promote fat burning, leading to long-term weight loss and improved health.

The benefits of regular exercise for weight loss and overall health

Regular exercise offers numerous benefits for weight loss and overall health. Exercise not only burns calories, but it also helps to increase metabolism, reduce body fat, improve cardiovascular health, and enhance mental well-being.

When it comes to weight loss, exercise can help to create a calorie deficit by burning calories and increasing the body's metabolic rate. Additionally, exercise can help to build muscle, which can increase metabolism and help to burn more calories at rest.

Types of exercise and their impact on metabolism

There are many types of exercise, including cardiovascular exercise (such as running, cycling, or swimming), strength training (using weights or resistance bands), and flexibility and balance exercises (such as yoga or pilates). Each type of exercise has a different impact on metabolism:

Cardiovascular exercise: Cardiovascular exercise, also known as aerobic exercise, can help to increase heart rate and breathing rate, burn calories, and improve cardiovascular health. This type of exercise can also help to increase metabolism both during and after exercise.

Strength training: Strength training can help to build muscle mass, which can increase metabolism and help to burn more calories at rest. In addition, strength training can also help to improve bone density and prevent muscle loss associated with aging.

Flexibility and balance exercises: Flexibility and balance exercises, such as yoga or pilates, can help to improve flexibility, balance, and posture. While these types of exercise do not burn as many calories as cardiovascular or strength training, they can still contribute to overall health and well-being.

Regular exercise is essential for weight loss and overall health. Cardiovascular exercise, strength training, and flexibility and balance exercises each offer unique benefits for metabolism and overall health. By incorporating a variety of exercises into a regular exercise routine, individuals can improve metabolism, burn more calories, and achieve and maintain a healthy weight.

Tips for designing an effective exercise program

Designing an effective exercise program is essential for achieving fitness goals and improving overall health. Here are some tips for designing an effective exercise program:

Set realistic goals: Set achievable and measurable goals that are specific to your needs and fitness level. Consider factors such as time, frequency, and intensity when setting goals.

Choose exercises that you enjoy: Choose exercises that you enjoy and that fit your lifestyle. This can help to increase motivation and adherence to the exercise program.

Gradually increase intensity: Gradually increase the intensity of your exercise program over time. This can help to prevent injury and improve overall fitness.

Include a variety of exercises: Incorporate a variety of exercises into your program, including cardiovascular exercise, strength training, and flexibility and balance exercises.

Rest and recover: Allow time for rest and recovery between exercise sessions. This can help to prevent injury and improve performance.

The importance of movement and staying active throughout the day

In addition to a structured exercise program, it's also important to stay active throughout the day. Sedentary behavior, such as sitting for long periods of time, can have negative effects on health, including increased risk of obesity, diabetes, and heart disease. Here are some tips for staying active throughout the day:

Take breaks: Take breaks from sitting every 30 minutes to stand up, stretch, and move around.

Walk or bike to work: If possible, walk or bike to work instead of driving.

Use the stairs: Use the stairs instead of the elevator or escalator whenever possible.

Incorporate activity into daily tasks: Incorporate activity into daily tasks, such as gardening or cleaning.

Stand while working: Consider using a standing desk or taking breaks to stand while working.

In summary, designing an effective exercise program and staying active throughout the day are both important for achieving fitness goals and improving overall health. By incorporating a variety of exercises into a structured program and staying active throughout the day, individuals can improve metabolism, burn more calories, and achieve and maintain a healthy weight.

Chapter 4: Lifestyle Factors

The Importance of Sleep, Stress Management, and Mindfulness

The importance of sleep, stress management, and mindfulness cannot be overstated when it comes to overall health and weight management.

Sleep: Sleep is essential for proper functioning of the body and mind. Lack of sleep can lead to increased stress, decreased energy levels, and impaired cognitive function. Studies have also shown that insufficient sleep is associated with an increased risk of obesity, diabetes, and other chronic health conditions. Therefore, it is important to prioritize getting enough quality sleep each night for optimal health and weight management.

Stress Management: Chronic stress can have negative effects on both physical and mental health. It can lead to overeating, poor food choices, and a decrease in physical activity, all of which can contribute to weight gain. Managing stress through techniques such as exercise, meditation, or mindfulness can help to reduce the negative impact of stress on the body and improve overall health.

Mindfulness: Mindfulness is the practice of being fully present and engaged in the present moment. It has been shown to have numerous health benefits, including reducing stress, improving cognitive function, and increasing overall well-being. When it comes to weight management, mindfulness can help to increase awareness of hunger and fullness cues, reduce emotional eating, and improve food choices.

Incorporating healthy sleep habits, stress management techniques, and mindfulness practices into daily life can have a positive impact on overall health and weight management. By prioritizing these aspects of self-care, individuals can improve their ability to manage stress, regulate their appetite and food choices, and ultimately achieve and maintain a healthy weight.

The role of sleep in weight loss and overall health

The role of sleep in weight loss and overall health:

Sleep plays a crucial role in weight loss and overall health. During sleep, the body performs important functions such as repairing and regenerating tissues, consolidating memories, and regulating hormones. Hormones such as leptin and ghrelin, which are involved in regulating appetite and metabolism, are also affected by sleep. Lack of sleep can disrupt these hormonal processes, leading to increased appetite, decreased energy expenditure, and weight gain.

Furthermore, insufficient sleep has been linked to an increased risk of chronic health conditions such as obesity, diabetes, and cardiovascular disease. To support weight loss and overall health, it is recommended to aim for 7-9 hours of quality sleep each night.

Understanding stress and its impact on weight

Stress is a natural response to a perceived threat or challenge. In the short term, stress can be beneficial, but when experienced chronically, it can have negative effects on physical and mental health, including weight gain.

Stress triggers the release of cortisol, a hormone that can increase appetite and cause the body to store fat, particularly around the midsection. Additionally, stress can lead to emotional eating, where individuals turn to food as a way to cope with stress or other negative emotions.

To manage stress and support weight loss, it is important to develop healthy coping mechanisms such as exercise, meditation, or mindfulness. Engaging in regular physical activity can also help to reduce stress and improve overall mood and well-being. Additionally, seeking support from friends, family, or a mental health professional can help to address underlying causes of stress and promote overall health and weight management.

Mindfulness and its role in healthy eating and weight loss

Mindfulness is a state of being fully present and engaged in the present moment without judgment. It has been shown to have numerous benefits, including improved mental health, reduced stress and anxiety, and increased overall well-being. When it comes to healthy eating and weight loss, mindfulness can play an important role in improving food choices, regulating appetite, and reducing emotional eating.

Mindful eating involves paying attention to the sensory experience of food, such as taste, smell, and texture. It also involves paying attention to hunger and fullness cues, as well as emotions and other factors that can influence eating habits. By being fully present and aware while eating, individuals can make more intentional and satisfying food choices, and avoid overeating or emotional eating.

Practicing mindfulness outside of meal times can also support healthy eating and weight loss. For example, mindfulness meditation or yoga can help to reduce stress and improve overall well-being, which can lead to improved food choices and weight management.

Other lifestyle factors that impact weight, such as smoking and alcohol consumption

Other lifestyle factors that impact weight, such as smoking and alcohol consumption, can also have negative effects on overall health and weight management. Smoking can lead to increased inflammation, decreased metabolic rate, and decreased physical activity, all of which can contribute to weight gain. Alcohol consumption, particularly excessive consumption, can lead to increased calorie intake, decreased inhibitions around food choices, and a disruption in sleep patterns, all of which can contribute to weight gain.

To support weight loss and overall health, it is important to adopt a holistic approach that includes healthy eating habits, regular exercise, adequate sleep, stress management, and mindful practices. Reducing or eliminating smoking and excessive alcohol consumption can also have positive effects on overall health and weight management. By prioritizing these lifestyle factors, individuals can support long-term weight loss and overall well-being.

Chapter 5: Setting Goals and Staying Motivated

Setting achievable goals and tracking progress is an important part of weight loss and weight management. Goals should be specific, measurable, achievable, relevant, and time-bound (SMART), and should be based on individual needs and preferences. By setting realistic goals and tracking progress, individuals can stay motivated and track their success over time.

To stay motivated and overcome obstacles, it is important to identify personal motivators and potential barriers to success. For example, individuals may find it helpful to identify their personal reasons for wanting to lose weight, such as improving overall health, increasing energy levels, or feeling more confident in their appearance. They can also identify potential barriers to success, such as a lack of time for exercise, emotional eating habits, or social pressures to overeat.

To overcome obstacles and stay motivated, individuals can try a variety of strategies, such as setting small, achievable goals, finding an accountability partner, seeking support from a healthcare provider or counselor, practicing self-compassion, and rewarding themselves for progress.

Strategies for maintaining weight loss and avoiding relapse include incorporating healthy habits into daily life, such as regular exercise and mindful eating, continuing to track progress, setting new goals, and seeking support from a healthcare provider or support group. It is also important to anticipate and prepare for potential challenges, such as holidays, social events, or periods of stress, and to have a plan in place for how to manage these situations without compromising progress.

Ultimately, maintaining weight loss and overall health requires a long-term commitment to healthy habits and a willingness to adapt and adjust as needed. By setting achievable goals, tracking progress, staying motivated, and adopting strategies for maintaining success, individuals can achieve sustainable weight loss and improve their overall well-being.